# Vibrational Nutrition for the New Era

# Vibrational Nutrition for the New Era

*by*

## Artimia Arian

TASHIRAT COSMIC LEARNING CENTER
TEPOZTLAN, MEXICO

www.Tashirat.com

Vibrational Nutrition for the New Era

Tashirat Learning Center, Tepoztlan, Mexico

For information address:
www.Tashirat.com
tashiratmail@gmail.com

*However, feel free to quote this book liberally, sharing the knowledge with as many people as possible. Please make the book available to anyone and everyone, anywhere and everywhere, in the hope that more humans on Planet Earth transform, becoming Human Beings, the Human connecting with and being guided by the Greater Self (or Being). The most efficient way to advertise and disseminate this knowledge is by transforming yourself, raising your vibration and becoming everything you always dreamed of but never thought possible.

The medical and health procedures in this book are based on the research, training and personal experience of the author. As each one of us and each situation is unique, the reader is urged to check with a qualified health professional when in doubt, before applying any procedure, and preferably to work under his / her supervision.

ISBN: 978-1-304-63159-6 (Pbk)

Cover & Back Photos by Thyesha Arian

# Acknowledgement and Dedication

*I thank God, the Divine Father of the All, and His remarkable Cosmic Doctors and Masters who have worked with me for the past fifteen years, enlightening me with this knowledge, enabling me to share it with humanity.*

*I dedicate this book to: all health practitioners and healers with New Era consciousness; to all suffering people with chronic or degenerative ailments vibrationally sensitive enough to be receptive to Integral Medicine; and to spiritual aspirants undergoing vibrational ascension.*

*In Truth, Love and Life,*
*Artimia Arian*

# Note to the Reader

This book is replete with knowledge that takes the reader's cosmic consciousness for granted. In addition, it can only be understood if the following books by Artimia Arian are read in the order presented:

**Cosmic Reawakening**

**Vibrational Nutrition**

**A Cosmic Understanding of Disease and Cure**

**Timeless Spiritual Teachings**

**Inspirational Quotes for the New Era**

**Essential Teachings for the New Era**

**Spiritual Vision for the New Era**


*For supplemental information please also read:*

**To Life!**

**Chakra Recipe Guide**

**The Tashirat Recipe Manual**

*For convenience, the masculine has been utilized not the feminine and they have not been used alternately as was done in some of my other books. No preference of sex is intended.*

*In Truth, Love and Life,*
*Artimia Arian*

# Table of Contents

A Note from the Author.................................... 1

Introduction............................................... 3

The Components of the Human Body.................. 9

The Chemical Elements of the Human Body....... 11

Correct Nutrition for the Cosmic Era................. 15

The Monumental Significance of
Dr. Robert Young's Work................................. 25

Lethal Digestive Ailments ................................ 31

Food Transitioning for Chakras 4 to 7.............. 35

Protein ........................................................ 37

Carbohydrates .............................................. 43

Blended Foods for Easy Digestion..................... 45

The New Era.................................................. 51

# A Note from the Author

*What I have termed Integral Medicine, is a comprehensive system combining Naturopathy (Natural Nutrition and Therapies – see Cosmic Reawakening), Homeopathy (a Vibrational Medicine system), and Cosmic Medicine. Cosmic Medicine is a Vibrational Medicine specifically suited to and vital for this New Era, with the Earth's vibration ascending. It encompasses all of the following: the individual's past evolution; present vibration; chakra life lessons mastered in this and past lifetimes; those yet to be mastered in this life time, and how to master them; the individual's vital force and constitutional strength; and the strength and balance of each of the primary chakras. In Integral Medicine, symptoms are explained and alleviated if necessary, but not suppressed. The student will learn and comprehend the root cause of disease in general and his/her condition in particular. The assimilation of the knowledge transmitted in one of my books, Cosmic Reawakening, is a pre-requisite for a full comprehension of the knowledge provided in this book.*

*The writing of cosmic books never takes more than one month (Cosmic Reawakening included). It's the experiential living and extensive experimentation required in perfecting this living experience, which converts a wealth of information into treasured confirmed knowledge, that takes years. The Nutrition knowledge in this book took years of toil to accumulate and for anyone ascending, or for patients with physical problems, the gems of essence knowledge delineated here, will be appreciated. For the successful treatment of patients in this era, in addition to the successful guidance of ascending spiritual aspirants, a thorough knowledge (self-lived) of Vibrational Nutrition is a fundamental necessity.*

1

*This is not intended to be a comprehensive Nutrition Manual. I have mostly provided essence Cosmic Knowledge, which is not found in other books. Wide collateral reading is a necessity, to supplement this knowledge. To practice Integral Medicine, a thorough knowledge of biochemical Nutrition is essential, as is a knowledge of Anatomy and Physiology, and Pathology and Disease. For Nutrition, the following books are highly recommended: Dr. Robert Young's Sick and Tired, and The pH Miracle; the Ann Wigmore books; the Norman Walker books, in particular Vegetable Juices; and The Chemistry of Man by Dr. Bernard Jensen. The School of Homeopathy in England, provides two outstanding correspondence courses in Anatomy and Physiology, and Pathology and Disease (in addition to superb Homeopathy courses).*

*It is important to understand that the perfect vibration is neither a high nor a low vibration. It is the exact vibration that the body requires at the time to balance its energies. Providing the perfect vibration with food (or Homeopathy or an energy cure) will result in a nearly instantaneous physical and/or emotional body fix (sometimes as rapid as fifteen minutes). Providing an imperfect vibration can result in digestive problems, nausea or emotional irritability and unhappiness.*

# *Introduction*

*A proper diet is probably the most important factor to consider during the treatment of any chronic illness. At least 90% of human ailments are traceable to faulty and inadequate nutrition. Almost every chronic disorder is related to an improper diet to a certain extent, and any permanent recovery cannot be expected if diet improvements are not adhered to. A sufficient supply of quality food is the most powerful of all curative agents. Food must be our first medicine and nutritional therapy the foremost therapy. Homeopathy, acupuncture, chiropractic adjustments, osteopathic work, herbal support, surgery, physical therapy, massage, yoga therapy and all other healing arts have their rightful place, but no healing can be successful without adequate nutritional support for patients. Only foods build, strengthen and repair damaged tissue. It is strange that in no field of study and observation has medical need been more insufficiently met than in that of nutrition, both in relation to the maintenance of health and to the treatment of disease.*

*It is important to realize that proper elimination of the body's waste is essential for health. Denatured foods cause slow starvation, while lack of elimination, due to a deficiency of alkaline elements (vegetables), causes acidosis or toxemia. Death through retention of waste poisons in the cells comes faster than death through starvation, because the fluids of the body must be alkaline to carry on the life processes.*

*Our bodies are composed of water, mineral salts, trace elements, proteins, glucides, lipids and vitamins. To function properly, the human body must be constantly replenished with foods that provide the aforementioned. The more live food one consumes the better, as cooking food destroys most of the enzymes and vitamins, and converts minerals into an inorganic unbalanced state.*

*On the chemical level, the body is composed of twenty-one essential chemical elements or minerals and each plays a special role. If the mineral salts required for blood and tissues are not provided in sufficient amounts, or if one of them is missing, health can decline rapidly. If appropriate cooking methods are not used, most of these minerals are destroyed or become impossible to assimilate.*

*These are the <u>eleven primary chemical elements which compose the human body</u> (and are therefore needed by the human body from food sources for proper functioning): Oxygen, carbon, hydrogen, nitrogen, sulfur (the soft tissue builders); calcium, phosphorus, magnesium (the bone builders); potassium, sodium, chlorine (electrolytes).*

*<u>The body's essential trace elements are</u>: Iron, copper, cobalt (along with oxygen are the blood builders); fluorine, zinc, silicon, iodine, selenium, manganese, molybdenum, chromium.*

*<u>The non-essential but useful trace elements are</u>: Vanadium, tin, nickel, arsenic, boron, strontium, lithium, germanium. There are about eighty-seven trace minerals in all.*

*<u>Acidifying foods are</u>: Refined and processed products, meat, junk food and overcooked or fried foods are acidifying. Meat and other cooked foods putrefy in the intestines and saturate the entire body. This causes the blood to become saturated with waste, which clogs the capillaries, causes painful congestion, and leads to the self-poisoning of the cells. An acidifying diet, deprived of its alkaline components, cannot neutralize the fermentation acids or the stomach acids.*

*Blood is the life of the body. In order to be fully efficient, the body must have 25 trillion perfect, round, disc-shaped red blood cells. The role of the red blood cells and plasma is to carry nutrients and oxygen to all parts of the body and transport used blood cells and*

4

*other toxic matter to the organs that will eliminate them. Many naturopaths agree that meat and other cooked foods that ferment in the digestive tract produce toxins, which cause these round discs to degenerate and be transformed into altered lifeless corpuscles that are exhausted and ready to expire.*

*Fruits and vegetables, when combined with nuts and seeds and raw food grains and other sprouts, are excellent sources of mineral salts. Since these foods do not produce fermentation or putrefaction after a short period in the digestive tract, they are obviously the appropriate foods for treating illnesses and preventing them.*

*Natural foods favor all the natural bodily functions. They keep the stomach clean, foster intestinal peristalsis, eliminate intestinal poisons and rid the body of the dangerous toxic waste that could cause pathological states in different body parts. This is the reason why a natural food diet is the essential basic principle in recovering and maintaining good health.*

*Our bodies are elaborated from the chemical elements that make up the soil of our planet. We must know and use foods that have the right chemical elements needed to sustain health. If your intake of minerals is below a certain amount, you will experience deficiency symptoms, and if your intake is above a certain amount, you will experience toxic effects. Body chemistry teaches you how and why you need certain amounts of nutrients and food chemistry teaches you the best food sources for those nutrients. A chemically balanced body is a healthy body. It is undeniable that for optimal health we also need exercise, fresh air, enough rest, recreation and a positive mental attitude which is usually related to a philosophical or spiritual vision.*

*Some individual's naturally absorb or assimilate larger quantities of certain biochemical elements. Their affinity for particular elements creates physical, mental and spiritual characteristics, which express and reflect the properties of those dominant biochemical patterns. Different people, due to inherent temperament, past evolution, metabolic disposition, mental activity, predominant faculties, and vibrational frequency, use the basic chemical elements at different rates, producing chemical imbalances in the body, which correspond to distinct types of temperament.*

*Dr. V.G. Rocine discovered a relationship between biochemical excesses or deficiencies and the basic human temperament type. Dr. V.G. Rocine was a Norwegian homeopath who claimed that excess or deficiency in any of the primary chemical elements needed in human nutrition could account for most diseases and psychopathic mental symptoms known to man. Thus, Rocine believed that food (along with essentials such as fresh air, sunshine, rest, etc.) was man's best medicine. Rocine believed that there was no such thing as a normal metabolism. Everyone is imbalanced in some respect, due to a faster or slower rate of utilization of one or more of the main chemical elements in the body. Personally I believe it is because of each individual's different rate of vibration, which is due to his evolution.*

*Dr. Rocine describes a calcium type, a silicon type of person, and types corresponding to many of the other elements so important in human nutrition. In the calcium type, there is a greater need for calcium foods in order for that person to express his or her particular temperament (more of a kundalini temperament), and if a calcium deficiency develops, not only is the body affected but the soul. The same principle follows for each of the chemical types of people. Thus for example, a phosphorus type would exhibit the qualities corresponding to the mineral element phosphorus. However, the person may possess an abundance of phosphorus in his body, either because he has a natural affinity to phosphorus-containing foods and eats them in excess or because he tends to absorb that mineral more than others. In either case it is because of the vibrational affinity between the individual and the mineral.*

*However, the person may burn that mineral faster than it can be replenished. A good example is the phosphorus cerebral person, who uses the mind and intellect but whose mental activities consume him. In such a case, even though he is clearly a phosphorus type, he could be deficient in the mineral and needs to consume larger quantities of that particular mineral, because of his predominantly mental and/or spiritual activities.*

*Therefore deficiencies always affect the body, soul and spirit. However, mineral deficiencies can be related to one's chakra balances or imbalances. Man is a spirit who lives in a body and has a soul. The spirit encourages the soul to develop its attributes and express them through the activities of the body.*

*We must learn to use food as a basis for correcting biochemical and vibrational deficiencies or imbalances, which affect mental as well as physical health. Mental, emotional and spiritual faculties can be changed by balancing the body biochemically and vibrationally through food.*

*Positivity is enhanced by certain elements – silicon, oxygen, iron, carbon, phosphorus, manganese and magnesium. Positivity and evolution are also enhanced by living one's correct chakra life lesson experience. Even if one's diet is optimal, without taking into account the correct chakra life experience of the person, health, which is balance, will be unattainable. A positive optimistic person expresses joy, hope, laughter, ideals, goals, love, social tendencies and deep emotions. These qualities contribute to increasing trust in humanity, eagerness for the future, a hopeful outlook on life, clearly defined personal life goals, positive mental attitudes and an active participation in living. Conversely, a lack of these expressions leads to negativity and pessimism. A strong influence of the following elements: nitrogen, calcium, fluorine, and chlorine, in addition to strong will faculties, strong reasoning faculties, commercial and self-preservation instincts (kundalini tendencies), will lead to the negative tendency outweighing the positive tendency.*

*Today we find many people relying on mineral supplements from the health food store, and although these have their place (due to depleted soil etc.), I believe we should get most of our minerals from foods. No chemical exits in isolation, except when prepared by laboratories. In nature, chemicals occur in groups – and we need these more complex forms in our bodies to ensure proper utilization and to avoid deficiencies. For example, without sufficient iodine and vitamin D, calcium cannot be properly used in the body; without vitamin B-12, iron cannot be assimilated. It is much more efficient and safe to get our minerals, vitamins and other nutrients from foods.*

*The cell salts needed for health are naturally triturated and potentized by plants in the process of photosynthesis. This raises the vibratory level of biochemicals to the point where they can be assimilated best by man. No human laboratory has yet learned to make foods better than Nature, or to improve upon Nature's methods. Foods bring in a sufficient variety of nutrients that the body can select what it needs, provided that we have sufficient variety in the diet.*

*Possessing a thorough knowledge of the body's components and constituent chemical elements, the minerals it requires for perfect functioning, the role these minerals play in the body, and their food sources, is rudimentary essential knowledge to all those who are interested in improving their own health and/or helping others to do the same. Possessing a thorough knowledge of the chakra life lessons and knowing the person's chakra strengths, weaknesses, balances or imbalances, and relating this to the chakra life lessons they need to zone in on, is equally essential to vibratory ascension and balancing, which in effect, is healing.*

# The Components of the Human Body

The human body is composed of (and must therefore be replenished by):

1. Water
2. Mineral Salts
3. Trace elements
4. Proteins
5. Glucides
6. Lipids
7. Vitamins

In living organisms there are two kinds of compounds: organic and inorganic. Organic compounds are composed of molecules that contain carbon atoms. Inorganic compounds generally do not contain carbon atoms (a few do). Organic molecules are generally larger and more complex than inorganic molecules. Both kinds of compounds are equally important to the chemistry of life.

The inorganic compounds of the body consist of: water and acids, bases and salts.

The major types of organic compounds found in the body are: carbohydrates, lipids (fats), proteins and nucleic acids.

Normally there are up to forty-six or more chemical elements that compose the human body. Five of them – carbon, hydrogen, oxygen, nitrogen and sulfur – make up ninety-nine percent of the body's molecules, mostly soft tissue and liquids (i.e. protein, carbohydrates, fats and water.)

*Chemical elements such as carbon, hydrogen, oxygen, nitrogen and sulfur, when joined together into large molecules become proteins, carbohydrates and fats.*

*Vitamins are needed for normal growth, tissue maintenance, and metabolism. They also work with enzymes to ensure that all the body's activities are carried out properly. Vitamins and minerals are called micronutrients because they are only needed in small amounts. Because most are not made by the body, they must be obtained from the diet. As with other nutrients, a deficiency of just one vitamin can cause problems for the entire body.*

*There is no substitute for the vitamins obtained from live foods. Like enzymes, many vitamins are destroyed in the cooking process. In addition, vitamins in live foods are often naturally combined with other nutrients for maximum absorption and used by the body. This is not something that can be duplicated in vitamin pills.*

*A person weighing 165 pounds carries about 115 lbs. of water, mostly in organic form although some is free. Saliva consists of 99% water, blood 80% and muscles 75%. Organic and inorganic compounds (both chemical and biochemical) are suspended in water solution, enhancing assimilation of building material into the blood; then worn-out material is expelled through the same medium. Tissue fluidity, elasticity, pliability and consistency are in direct proportion to the amount of water contained in that tissue.*

*Consumption of distilled water in large quantities washes waste products and toxins from the body, destroys germs and cleanses the organism (with the aid of chlorine); but the prolonged usage of distilled water is not advised because it also draws mineral salts from the body. It is more indicated in cases of arthritis, hardening and deposits in the body. Vegetable juices are the best source of organic water and they are minerally-rich.*

# The Chemical Elements of the Human Body

*The fundamental purpose of eating is to replenish the chemical elements composing the cells and tissues in our body. Here is an outline of the chemical elements in an average adult body and where these elements can be found in the body.*

## The Adult Human Body

*The Human Body is composed on an average of the following atomic elements*

| Element | Approx. % | In the formation mainly of |
|---------|-----------|----------------------------|
| Oxygen | 65 | Bones, Teeth, Skin, Red blood corpuscles, Circulation, Optimism |
| Carbon | 18 | Teeth, Connective Tissue, Skin, Hair, Nails |
| Hydrogen | 10 | Blood and all the Cells in the body |
| Nitrogen | 3 | Muscles, Cartilage, Tissues, Ligaments, Tendons, lean flesh |
| Calcium | 2 | Bones and Teeth |
| Phosphorus | 1 | Blood and Brain |
| Potassium | 0.4 | Blood, Bones and all Cells |

| | | |
|---|---|---|
| Sulfur | 0.25 | Blood |
| Sodium | 0.25 | Skin, Nerves, Mucous Membrane |
| Chlorine | 0.25 | Epithelium, Nerves, etc. |
| Fluorine | 0.2 | Nails, Hair, Blood, Skin |
| Magnesium | 0.05 | Blood, Nerves, Muscles |
| Iron | 0.008 | Blood, Bones, Brain, Muscles, etc. |
| Manganese | 0.003 | Hemoglobin, Lymph, etc. |
| Silicon | 0.0002 | Blood, Muscles, Nerves, Skin, Hair, Nails |
| Iodine | 0.00004 | Thyroid, Blood, Spinal Nerves, Brain, Bone, Metabolism |

*(Taken from Diet and Salad by Dr. N.W. Walker, D.Sc.)*

*Our vital organs, glands, bones, ligaments, muscles, and other tissues of the body each have their own special nutritional needs. The following table lists the specific chemical element needed by each tissue type.*

| Tissue Type | Nutrient |
|---|---|
| Adrenals | Zinc |
| Blood | Iron |
| Bowel | Magnesium |
| Brain/Nerves | Phosphorus/Oxygen |
| Heart | Potassium/Magnesium |
| Kidneys | Chlorine |
| Liver | Iron/Sulfur |

| Lungs | Silicon |
|---|---|
| Muscles | Potassium |
| Hair/Nails | Silicon |
| Pituitary | Phosphorus |
| Skin | Silicon/Sulfur |
| Spleen | Copper/Chlorine |
| Stomach | Sodium/Chlorine |
| Teeth/Bones | Calcium/Fluoride |
| Thyroid | Iodine |

*(Taken from Guide to Body Chemistry and Nutrition by Dr. Bernard Jensen)*

*In greater detail:*

# The Body and the Chemical Elements

*Body proteins:* Carbon, hydrogen, oxygen, nitrogen plus phosphorus, sulfur and iron in many cases.
*Body fat:* Carbon, hydrogen, oxygen.
*Required for cell metabolism:* Iron, phosphorus, sodium, potassium, calcium, magnesium, sulfur, manganese, copper.
*Percentage of water in tissues:* Fat – 20%, blood – 80%, bone – 25%, kidneys – 80%, liver – 70%, muscle – 75%, skin 70%, brain 85%, nerves -70%.
*Muscle:* Potassium, magnesium, chlorine, manganese, calcium, phosphorus, selenium.
*Bones and teeth:* Calcium, phosphorus, magnesium, fluorine, silicon, copper, manganese.
*Joints and ligaments:* Sodium, iron, manganese.
*Hair and nails:* Silicon, iron, sulfur, zinc, chlorine.
*Skin:* Silicon, sulfur, sodium, manganese, copper.
*Brain and nervous system:* Phosphorus, magnesium, potassium, sodium, iodine, sulfur, silicon, calcium, manganese.

_Heart:_  Magnesium, iron, potassium, calcium, phosphorus.
_Blood:_  Iron, copper, zinc, sodium, potassium, calcium.
_Blood vessels:_  Magnesium, silicon, sulfur.
_Spleen:_  Iron, copper, fluorine, sodium, potasssium, magnesium.
_Liver:_  Zinc, selenium, sulfur, iron, potassium, magnesium.
_Kidneys:_  Potassium, chlorine, fluorine, manganese, magnesium, calcium, iron, silicon.
_Lungs:_  Phosphorus, manganese, silicon.
_Gastrointestinal system:_  Sodium, potassium, chlorine, fluorine, iodine, calcium, iron.
_Anus:_  Silicon.
_Bladder:_  Silicon, fluorine.
_Inner ear:_  Magnesium, fluorine, iron, chlorine.
_Eyes:_  Sulfur, fluorine.
_Pituitary:_  Iodine, phosphorus, sulfur, manganese, bromine.
_Pineal:_  Phosphorus, sulfur, manganese.
_Adrenal medulla:_  Phosphorus, sulfur, manganese, iodine.
_Adrenal cortex:_  Calcium, fluorine, iron, silicon.
_Thyroid, parathyroid, thymus:_  Sodium, potassium, chlorine, magnesium, iodine.
_Pancreas, Islets of Langerhans:_  Zinc, manganese, potassium, chromium.
_Prostate:_  Zinc, silicon, magnesium.
_Testes, ovaries:_  Silicon, manganese, magnesium, phosphorus, zinc.

_(Taken from The Chemistry of Man By Bernard Jensen, Ph.D)_

# Correct Nutrition for the Cosmic Era

*The word "basic" is derived from the Greek "basis," meaning foundation. In a chemical sense, the word relates to the properties of acidity and alkalinity. When a metal ion is with a hydroxyl ion, we have a base, and when a hydrogen ion is with a negative ion such as chloride or sulphate, we have an acid. The term "alkali" means the same as soda ash, and alkali metals such as sodium and potassium make strong bases. When these bases engage with acids, there is a chemical warfare between them that ends in a chemical salt. A base turns litmus paper blue, while an acid will turn it red. Acids and bases are chemical opposites.*

*The human body is not the same as a chemist's laboratory. The human body is complex, with acids, bases, enzymes, heat, fermentation etc., with the emotions capable of shifting the chemical environment at any moment. Foods that are basic in the laboratory may not be in the stomach, nor will they respond the same in the digestive tracts of different people. That which neutralizes acidity in one stomach may not do so in another.*

*The most alkaline food element is sodium, followed by magnesium. Food potassium is alkaline to the muscles and urinary system. Calcium is alkaline to the bones, magnesium to the nerves. Manganese is alkaline to the brain, and iron to blood. Sodium is alkaline to the alimentary tract. The alkaline principle in foods can cure most diseases.*

*A diet based on alkalizing vegetables, sprouted and soaked nuts and seeds, essential oils, and low-sugar fruits will restore health, harmony and balance. Normalizing the blood and tissue pH will reduce the amount of symptom-causing microforms in the body and thereby reduce symptoms.*

*Robert Young is able to analyze your blood and describe to you your symptoms. He reports, "The thousands of blood samples I've studied from all over the world reveal the amazing cellular changes that occur with diet changes. As a person eats more alkalizing foods, especially raw vegetables and greens, I see extreme improvement in red blood cell integrity, oxygenation of the blood, and levels of negative microforms." (The pH Miracle).*

*All food digested in our bodies metabolizes or burns down to an ash residue, which can be neutral, acidic or alkaline, mostly depending on the mineral content of the original food. Potassium, calcium, magnesium, sodium, zinc, silver, copper, and iron form alkaline ash; sulfur, phosphorus, chlorine, and iodine leave acid ash. Most elements are alkaline.*

*"It is easy to categorize which foods leave what kind of ash. In general, animal foods – meat, eggs, dairy – processed and refined foods, yeast products, fermented foods, grains, artificial sweeteners, fruit, and sugars are acidifying, as are alcohol, coffee, chocolate, black tea, and sodas. Vegetables, on the other hand, are alkalizing. That includes a few that are technically fruits: avocado, tomato, bell pepper. A few nonsweet citrus fruits are also basic in the body, as are sprouted seeds, nuts, and grains. Grains are acidifying, though a few (millet, buckwheat, and spelt) are only very mildly so. Raw foods are more alkalizing, while cooked food is more acidifying." (The pH Miracle, Robert Young).*

*Young advocates that in order to maintain a balanced pH in the blood and tissues, the diet should consist of at least 70-80% alkaline (or basic) foods.*

## Vegetables

*Chlorophyll helps the blood cells deliver oxygen throughout the body. Leafy greens have the highest amount of chlorophyll. Green vegetables are also high in chlorophyll. Vegetables and especially green vegetables, are exceedingly nutrient-packed and provide just about all the vitamins, minerals, and micronutrients the body could ever need. Vegetables are also extremely high in fiber, which is crucial to the diet. Fiber not only aids the peristaltic movement, studies have demonstrated that they markedly decrease mycotoxicity. The fibers act like a sponge, soaking up acids from the body. Fibers are the best brooms, cleaning out the intestines.*

*Vegetables, especially raw vegetables, have an abundance of enzymes required for nearly every chemical operation in the body. Among other things, enzymes aid digestion. By eating live foods replete with enzymes, one boosts one's overall enzyme potential and therefore one's overall energy level, because whatever the enzymes in the food could accomplish in the way of digestion, makes less work for the digestive enzymes in the body. The body can rather make more metabolic enzymes for other functions such as repairs associated with mycotoxin damage.*

*Tomatoes and avocados are good vegetable choices (technically they are fruits), because eaten raw, they are alkalizing and low in sugar. They have more potassium than bananas and far less sugar.*

## Grains

*Wheat and rice are the most acid-forming grains (they create mucus too). Amaranth, quinoa, and spelt are slightly acidic, and millet and buckwheat are more neutral and do not provoke mucus formation. They are also high in protein and digest slowly, thus keeping the blood sugar balanced.*

## Protein

Non-animal protein can be provided from tofu, legumes, raw nuts, sprouted seeds and grains, avocados. These are all high-quality proteins that are better assimilated than animal proteins. All the rest of the proteins the body needs can be acquired from greens. The key to providing the body with protein is quality, not quantity.

The body has a free amino acid pool, which contributes about seventy grams of protein daily. Most people have protein reserves. Unless you have specific protein deficiency symptoms (muscle tissue loss, hair falling out, brittle nails), you don't have to worry, you are getting enough protein. Vegetables carry all the amino acids the body needs, as long as you are consuming a wide variety and supplementing with grasses.

Meat (pork, beef, lamb, chicken, turkey, etc.) and eggs are filled with hormones, pesticides, steroids, antibiotics, microforms, mycotoxins, and the saturated fats that contribute to heart disease, strokes and cancer, among other ailments. There is a strong correlation between animal protein and several kinds of cancer. Studies show that people who get 70% of their protein from animal products have major health difficulties compared to those who get a small percentage of their protein that way.

Besides, animal foods are dead in every respect, including lack of enzymes. Vegetable foods, alive with enzymes, energy, and phytonutrients, are far superior in every way. Whatever nutrients may be in animal foods, they simply are not worth the risks – not to mention the stress they put on the body during digestion and through the energy required to extract what nutrients they contain. All meats are permeated with microforms and their toxins. Most mycotoxins are heat-tolerant, so cooking doesn't get rid of them. Anatomically and physiologically, humans are not meant to be carnivores or omnivores.

18

*Vitamin B12*

*Many people base their criticism of vegetarianism on the dietary absence of the anti-pernicious vitamin B-12. They overlook the fact that this vitamin is heat sensitive and over 85% of its effectiveness can be lost under normal cooking conditions. Since no-one eats raw meat, people cannot make claim to animal protein as being a source of this vitamin. Then, the question has to be raised why are we not having a widespread planetary epidemic of pernicious anemia?*

*It has been revealed that the ultimate source of all vitamin B-12 is certain bacteria. It seems that vitamin B-12 needs of human and animal is adequately supplied by the intestinal tract bacteria.*

*The main causes of development of vitamin B-12 deficiency are as following:*
- *A thick coating of mucus and slime along the intestinal tract, which reduces permeability to all vitamins.*
- *Putrefactive bacteria predominate due to such factors as overeating, poor food combinations, high protein diet, excess sugar, smog, enzyme deficiency, insecticides.*

*The most pronounced symptom for vitamin B-12 deficiency is extreme sensitivity to heat and cold – normal tap water feels like ice, with pins and needle pain on the skin. The condition can be corrected within about two weeks by following good food combining, eating only when hungry, eliminating all sweets, cutting down on protein, and increasing the greens and sprouts in one's diet. Acidophilus/bifidus will help too. The putrefactive bacteria, with associated gas, will be replaced by friendly bacteria which are noted for the manufacture of the B-complex vitamins, including the B-12.*

*The following foods contain Vitamin B-12: eggs, milk and dairy products, dulse, kelp, soybeans and soy products, sunflower seeds, and alfalfa (the latter being a rare plant source of B-12).*

## Essential Fatty Acids

*EFAs are vital to good health and play many roles in the body. Polyunsaturated fats such as flax, borage, evening primrose, grape seed, and hemp oils help construct cell membranes, produce hormones, and bind and eliminate acids. Most oils contain both monounsaturated and polyunsaturated fats, and those that are predominately monounsaturated, such as olive oil, raw nuts and avocados, are used for cellular energy, (rather than sugars).*

## Sprouts

*Sprouts are full of vitamins, minerals and complete proteins. They are about the best food you can eat. Seeds become more alkaline as they sprout and sprouts are packed with enzymes. They are biogenic – they transfer their life energy to you. The following sprouts can be used: alfalfa sprouts, mung bean sprouts, chickpea sprouts, green lentil sprouts, sesame sprouts, sunflower sprouts, buckwheat sprouts, and wheat sprouts.*

## Carbohydrates (Sugars)

*Avoid sugar like the plague – it feeds negative microforms. Microforms love all forms of sugar (white, brown, processed beet, cane, corn sugars and syrups, maple syrup, honey, molasses, sucrose, fructose, maltose, lactose, glucose, mannitol, sorbitol, galactose, date sugar, and even natural sugars from fruit, especially those that cause a rapid rise in blood sugar.)*

*In any form microforms love sugar and will ferment it into alcohol and other mycotoxins and create an acidic environment in your body. Therefore though fruit has many good vitamins and* minerals, and is rich in fiber, it is also filled with sugar, so must be eaten in moderation only when the body is in balance. All the same nutritional benefits can be derived from vegetables, without the negative side effects.

Almost all fruits must be avoided until the body has returned to balance and then eat fruits in moderation. However lemons, lime and non-sweet grapefruit are beneficial. Fruit is nutrient-rich and healthy, but the sugar it contains ferments like any other sugar, and wreaks the familiar havoc in your system once it is already out of balance (most people). Lemons, limes and grapefruit are acid but have an alkalizing affect when they are metabolized in the body. They have very little sugar and contain an abundance of oxygen, which prevents microform overgrowth.

The high carbohydrate vegetables (potatoes, pumpkin, cooked peas and carrots) should be eaten in moderation.

### Dairy Products

Like most animal foods, dairy products contain hormone and pesticide residues, microforms, mycotoxins, and saturated fats. They also have lactose which breaks down like any sugar and feeds harmful microforms. All dairy foods are the most highly mucus-forming and acid-foods. Soy, nut and seed milks are far superior (best home-made as store bought products usually have sugar). The best dairy milk, if you are still transitioning, is unprocessed goat's milk from organically grown and grazing cows. It contains the antifungal caprylic acid.

Milk is designed for baby cows. What animal in nature consumes milk after infancy, and from another species? Cow's milk is far too concentrated for human consumption, and is ultra acidic in the bloodstream. Cow's milk contains three times the calcium, three times the protein, ten times the phosphorus, and three hundred times the amount of casein (one of the strongest glues used by *carpenters) found in human milk. We have a hard time trying to excrete all the excesses from cow's milk that our bodies cannot assimilate.*

*As far as calcium intake is concerned (the reason most mothers force their children to drink milk), one of the roles calcium plays in the body is to neutralize acids. When animal proteins are consumed, generating higher levels of acidity, greater quantities of calcium are required to neutralize the acidity. If you eat these acidic foods and the calcium available in the body falls short, calcium is withdrawn from the bones and teeth to try and return the body to an alkaline state. Many experts therefore blame osteoporosis on protein overdose. John Robbins in his book Diet for a New World, cites many studies relating to how calcium-rich dairy products actually leave the body with a negative calcium balance by the time all that protein is buffered.*

*To normalize a calcium deficiency, one needs to eat a flesh free, dairy free, low acid producing diet, so that normal quantities of calcium are required and all calcium ingested is optimally utilized. We are usually calcium deficient when a general mineral imbalance exists. Consuming 2 lts. of vegetable juices daily will rectify this problem, if accompanied by a healthy diet and lifestyle.*

*For a list of calcium-rich foods please refer to the section on calcium further on.*

<u>*Water and Vegetable Juice*</u>

*As important as what you eat is what you drink, and most of us don't drink enough. Our bodies are seventy percent water and drinking water of the highest quality is vital to health. Water is the vehicle for all exchanges in the body. The body requires a daily supply of 2-3 lts., depending on how much live food you consume (the more you consume, the less you will need to drink).*

22

*Sufficient hydration is essential to a clean body. Getting liberal amounts of alkaline water neutralizes stored acid wastes and, if consumed every day in conjunction with a good diet, removes the acids from the body. Two elements are necessary for the body to cleanse itself: plant fiber – to accelerate digestion and help form stools, and water – to help produce urine.*

*As we've seen, water is an inorganic compound. The only way in which it can become organic, or instilled with the life-principle, is through the vegetable kingdom. The chemicals of the mineral kingdom are dead and inorganic, but when dissolved by Nature and absorbed in plant life, or vegetation, then they become organized with the life principle and so become organic.*

*When fruits and vegetables are heated above 118∘F, the heat reconverts the organic chemicals back into their inorganic lifeless state. The same applies to water, whether it is from the tap, rain, spring or distilled, water is inorganic. However, when fed to vegetation, it is absorbed into the plant and becomes organic. The elements composing the original water are then separated and stored in the fibers of the plant.* **Therefore the raw juice from all fruits and vegetables is the finest organic water obtainable.** *In the extraction of this water, as juice, the chemicals that were in the vegetable or fruit are also present, and in this natural state these also are organic.*

*All the benefits of vegetables (and grasses) can be enhanced by juicing them. The nutrients are more concentrated and more quickly and easily available to the body. You do lose the fiber with juicing, but that is what frees the nutrients (chewing has the same effect, but it is not as effective as juicing.) When you drink your vegetables, your body is getting a greater concentration of rapidly usable alkaline salts, vitamins, minerals, chlorophyll, and enzymes. Vegetable juices are very alkalizing. They also have an important cleansing effect in the intestines.*

*The processes of digestion are vital processes in which organic water plays by far the most important part. The digestive juices themselves in the body are composed of more than 98% organic water. In their operation it is important that this organic water be constantly replenished.*

*Distilled water is best and if some fresh lemon juice is squeezed into it, it is tasty and alkalizing.*

\*\*\*\*\*\*\*\*\*\*\*\*\*\*\*\*\*\*\*\*\*\*\*\*\*\*\*\*\*\*\*\*\*\*\*\*\*\*\*\*\*\*\*\*\*\*

*Under the category Food Sources, when discussing each chemical element, I have not only included the above ideal foods, I have also included dairy products and acid-forming carbohydrates, for people who are still transitioning. I have excluded meat; fish is preferred if transitioning. Gradually transitioning from a diet of meat, sugar, heavily spiced foods, dairy products, processed and refined products, etc. to a healthy high percentage live food diet, helps the body and mind to gradually adapt and become purified.*

# The Monumental Significance of Dr. Robert Young's Work

(I do not personally know Dr. Robert O. Young, but from years of experience on ourselves, our Tashirat children and students, his research in the field of microbiology and nutrition has proved invaluable. If transitioned correctly, fully taking into consideration the person's vibration, evolution and present condition, we find the alkaline diet that Dr. Young prescribes not only healthy, but in many cases also life-saving.)

*In this chapter, I will briefly summarize Dr. Robert Young's theory, his emphasis on the importance of the blood pH being balanced and how food choices directly affect the body's pH balance more than any other factor. The following chapter describes an alkalizing diet. I have included both these chapters in order to explain the food sources I have selected for each mineral, in relation to learning how to balance the body's biochemistry.*

## About Dr. Robert Young

*Robert O. Young, Ph.D., D.Sc., (in Microbiology and Nutrition) has devoted his life to researching the causes of disease and helping people recuperate lost health. As a microbiologist, he has investigated the links between over-acidification of the body and the development of morbid microorganisms (bacteria, yeast, fungus, and mold), whose metabolic poisons produce the wide range of symptoms we generally call "diseases." He stresses the importance for correct acid-alkaline balance in the body, based on healthy lifestyle, diet, and nutritional supplementation. He has gained national recognition (he is an American) for his research into diabetes, cancer, leukemia, and AIDS. He is the author of two superlative books – Sick and Tired and The pH Miracle.*

*I intend to only very briefly outline his theory, which is actually an extension of the collective academic wisdom of prominent researchers, but I urge anyone interested, to purchase his books. Many books are outstanding but few are life-transforming. These two books transformed my life and as I re-educated myself, the life of Tashirat staff, children, students and patients were equally transformed.*

## Dr. Robert Young's Theory

*Robert Young's general stance is no different to that of all Naturopaths or Alternative Medicine practitioners – an unbalanced terrain is what lies behind most, if not all, symptom pictures. In the early stages of the imbalance, the outer symptoms may not be very intense and are frequently treated with drugs. They include: skin eruptions, headaches, allergies, colds and flu, and sinus problems. As things progress, weakened organs and systems start to give way – thyroid, adrenals, liver, etc. Chronic diseases which later become degenerative, take hold if the root of the problem is not eradicated. There are no enemies or specific diseases to fight, simply the consequence of balance or imbalance of the internal terrain.*

*Dr. Young correctly maintains that germs seek their natural habitat – diseased tissue – rather than being the cause of the diseased tissue. Mosquitoes seek stagnant water. Rather than trying to kill every single mosquito, clean the water. Up until this point, there is nothing new in his theory.*

*To me, the following information was what expanded my consciousness and life. Robert Young proved (in Sick and Tired he provides countless microscope photographs to demonstrate his* *point) that when the environment is dirty, from inverted dietary and lifestyle habits, **any normal cell** (red or white blood cell, liver, kidney, brain cell) **can transform and rapidly change its form and function** (sometimes in a matter of minutes), **and become a bacteria, yeast or fungus.** In a process which is known as pleomorphism, he demonstrates photographically how bacteria can and do change into yeast, yeast into fungus, and fungus to mold.*

*So actually the one physiological disease is an acidic toxic terrain. Germs born out of this compromised terrain, are primary symptoms. The symptom or collection of symptoms that the germs provoke, are secondary symptoms (what traditional medicine commonly refers to as the various diseases).*

*Young's work is an extension of many researchers (Gunther Enderlein 1872-1968 and Antoine Bechamp 1816 -1908 are two of the most prominent), who likewise witnessed and therefore adhered to the principle of pleomorphism in their research. Pleomorphism literally means many forms. Microorganisms, such as a specific bacterium, can take on multiple forms, which is a change of function as well as shape.*

*There is a lost chapter is history that these aforementioned giants belong to, which reveals that there is something living independently in cells and body fluids which is capable of evolving into more complex forms. These independent life elements are known as microzymas (small beings). All living things contain them. **Degeneration and regeneration both originate with the microzymas.** All cells evolve from them to begin with. In the right circumstances and environment, microzymas evolve into more complex life forms, including bacteria and fungi. Bacteria can also devolve back to microzymas. Everything begins and ends with microzymas. What happens in between depends on the environment. These harmful pleomorphic organisms do not and* *cannot evolve in healthy alkaline terrain. In a healthy environment, microzymas build and work with the body.*

*These harmful microorganisms and their wastes contribute directly or indirectly to a huge list of symptoms. Most diseases, especially chronic and degenerative ones, are a result of microform overgrowth. Yeast and fungus overgrowths underlie condition such as AIDS, diabetes, hypoglycemia, cancer, atherosclerosis, osteoporosis, chronic fatigue and the list continues.*

***It is highly significant to note that pleomorphic changes can only be seen if you look at live blood, not by stained blood samples.*** *Robert Young used a high-powered light microscope, a video recorder, and a printer, to record the evolution of poleomorphic organisms from rod-shaped bacteria (bacilli) to spherical (cocci), and finally into yeast and fungus and mold – and back again. Apparently pleomorphism has also been seen in recent electron microscope pictures of animal tissue.*

*Microforms thrive in acidity. They also thrive in low oxygen levels that come with acidity and the wastes they produce are strong acids themselves. To reverse the process, all we have to do is alkalize our bloodstream. When the body goes from acid back to alkaline, yeast, fungus, and mold stop growing and revert to being benign. Their leftover toxins can then be bound up by certain fats and minerals and eliminated from the body. Germs are everywhere, but they can't grow and multiple and make you sick (or kill you) unless the environment is good for them – acidic!*

*Microform overgrowth is natural when life is ending. The body stops breathing, oxygen levels drop, creating the anaerobic environment microforms thrive in. They are designated to decompose our dead bodies. What is unnatural is that they start taking over overly acidic living bodies – the process is set in motion prematurely. They are not inherently bad in themselves, they are if anything good, serving as the garbage collectors who handle the recycling of cells which are constantly breaking down. We simply need to alkalize our terrain.*

*Overacidity and microform overgrowth are inextricably linked. Microforms are a major source of acid in the blood. We predispose ourselves to both conditions through various stresses. The main one is poor diet, although chronic toxicity from external sources and other physiological stresses such as poor digestion (also due to poor diet and dietary combinations), play roles too. Emotional trauma, negative thinking patterns and other psychological stress also contribute.*

*A vicious cycle of imbalance takes hold. First comes the initial stress (poor diet, negative thinking, spiritual distress, destructive emotions) which starts to acidify the body and disturb the cells. The cells work to adapt to the declining pH of their compromised environment. They break down and evolve to bacteria, yeast, fungus, and molds. These in turn create their waste products – debilitating acids – which further pollute the environment. It's a vicious cycle. According to Robert Young, most people have microform overgrowth.*

*To end on an optimistic note, Robert Young also discovered the following from his mind expanding research: red blood cells (non-nucleated) have the ability to de-evolve (dedifferentiate) into blastema cells (nucleated embryonic cells) and become (differentiate into) any cell needed by the body for regeneration e.g. red blood cells can become bone cells, muscle cells, skin cells, brain cells, heart cells, liver cells, etc. So depending on the state of the environment, red blood cells can regenerate or degenerate the body.*

*He defines a healthy or diseased terrain by determining primarily four factors:*
- *Its acid / alkaline balance (pH)*
- *Its electric / magnetic charge (negative or positive)*

- *Its level of poisoning (toxicity)*
- *Its nutritional status*

# Lethal Digestive Ailments

*Indigestion underlies most disease conditions and its symptoms. Recurrent or chronic digestive problems are lethal. Digestive problems create the perfect environment for negative bacteria, yeast and fungus to survive and proliferate, causing havoc in the body. It is important to realize that there are few pain receptor nerves in the bowel area, so it takes a severe problem to cause even minor discomfort. Because of this, gradual impediment of the large intestine especially (the colon or lower bowel), may pass unnoticed for years, until one day a really serious condition exists.*

*Our digestive tracts house large populations of bacteria, many of which are fundamental to our health. These are the intestinal flora or "friendly bacteria," without which we cannot live. The primary ways in which these friendly bacteria are abused are the following: wrong food, poor food combinations, medications (antibiotics, steroids, cortisone and all other allopathic medicated drugs), mental and emotional stress. All the above factors plus environmental pollution, injury, incorrect breathing and other factors, contribute to the development and evolution of Y/F as well as many other detrimental bacterial forms.*

*The colon easily becomes toxic because of its function in disposing of body wastes. It is the most heavily laden organ with toxic, drug or systemic settlements. This waste material often remains in the large intestine for months and even years, decaying more and more, producing poisons, and seeping into the body through the bowel wall, and entering the bloodstream, thus poisoning the entire system. Most of this seepage is gradual except in when the fungus actually perforates the bowel wall and penetrates into the blood stream.*

*If unfriendly bacteria and mycotoxin-producing organisms multiply prodigiously, eventually forming colonies, dysbiosis results. Dysbiosis is an imbalance in the intestinal micro-populations. When fungi colonize, they form tube-like structures which pierce the colon wall and the fungus enters directly into the bloodstream.*

*These perforations and their toxic channels can be clearly seen as dark lines radiating from the pupil or the autonomic nerve wreath (a circular ring a little away from the pupil). Where radii solaris or radial furrow signs are present in the iris, know that the seepage is no longer gradual. The darker the color of these lines or radii solari, as they are termed in iridology, the more chronic or degenerative the condition (the longer it has persisted). The more numerous the lines, the more body parts are affected. (The affected parts can easily be identified if you have but a basic knowledge of the iridology chart). Yeast and fungus always attack the body's weakest areas by poisoning and overworking them and by directly penetrating their cells.*

*If waste material is not regularly evacuated from the intestines, it will accumulate and the toxic products of decomposition may be taken up by the blood and lymph and be carried to every cell in the body. The intestinal tract is usually the beginning of toxic settlements found in all the other organs (this is so evident in the iris).*

*How does the colon become unclean? The digestive tract is protected by a clear slippery substance known as mucus. It protects the surface of the digestive tract membranes. Mucus is a healthy secretion and is secreted upon the ingestion of any material, even water. However, mucus has the additional function of engulfing toxins. The thick opaque mucus you are familiar with when you have a cold, is the result of the healthy transparent mucus engulfing toxins, in an attempt to remove them from the body. Mucoid-forming foods are therefore all foods that contain*

32

*toxins or alternatively foods that break down in such a way that they cause the intestine to produce mucus to trap these toxins. Dairy products, starches, and all denatured foods fall into this category. If these foods are consumed regularly over an extended period, the large intestine becomes encrusted with fecal-mucoid material and debris, thus promoting the growth of Y/F and other morbid microforms. Live vegetables are not at all mucoid-forming (other than the very sweet ones such as carrot, red pepper and beet, if you already have Y/F).*

*Poor food combining is also a chief cause of mucoid production as well as Y/F overgrowth. (Please refer to To Life! by Artimia Arian for food combining guidelines).*

*If the bowel is very toxic, the colon area in the left iris usually shows more toxicity than in the right. The reason for this is that as waste material passes through the large colon, it becomes dryer, as much fluid has been absorbed. If bowel movements are not regular there is a backing-up process and a greater amount of concentrated toxic material is found in the descending colon and in the sigmoid. This can be responsible for heart, ovarian and bladder troubles.*
*It is believed that disorders such as appendicitis, infected tonsils, liver and gall-bladder infections, dysfunction of heart and blood vessels, sinusitis, arthritis and rheumatism, etc., no doubt have their origin in a sluggish colon. There is also an increasing number of morbid conditions in the various parts of the colon, involving the flexures, the rectum, and the anus. Consider the amount of surgery and various therapies for hemorrhoids, fistulas, prostate disturbances, and malignancies.*

*The slower the movement of waste material through the colon, the greater the bacterial content and the greater the possibility of putrefaction. The time required for ridding the bowel of toxic material depends on how toxin free the bowel wall is. This can be determined by the extent to which toxic settlement is indicated in the iris. The older and more chronic it is, the slower it will move.*

*Accumulated matter in any disposal system, decays and omits foul odors when allowed to become stagnant. It is said that normal human feces consists chiefly of dead bacteria, millions being excreted daily.*

*The person who suffers from bowel constipation also has a type of tissue constipation and encumbrance in other parts of his body such as the eyes, gall bladder, liver, kidneys, lungs, etc. Constipation increases the work of other organs of excretion and may result in their depletion. Constipation is the root cause of most of the diseases today. There is usually no organ reflected in the iris that appears as dark as the bowel area. The bowel seems to be the center of importance in the body and when it is clean and in a healthy condition other organs are, as a rule, healthy. Every organ is dependent upon the intestinal tract. It is the center from which all organs extend. In constipation, toxic material accumulates and develops in the bowel, finally to be thrown off into the blood stream to escape in whatever manner it can. It may settle in the leg area, or it may be thrown into any organ of the body. When the liver and bowels are functioning better, symptoms begin to disappear and the patient feels better because new life and energy are now flowing through the vital organs.*

# Food Transitioning for Chakras 4 to 7

## Chakra 4

1. Lightly steamed lentil sprouts (5-10 mins.) or other sprouted legumes such as
garbanzos or soy beans.
2. All steamed vegetables; the green vegetables have higher vibrations and mineral contents (e.g. broccoli, Brussel sprouts, green beans, cabbage, zucchini with the skin, spinach or any other green leafy vegetable steamed for two minutes)
3. Steamed vegetables mixed with raw vegetables or with green leaves or sprouts to raise the meal's vibration.
4. Dehydrated vegetables and nut/seed crackers.

Both steamed and raw vegetables can be eaten with seaweed or avocado (both Ch. 3) or with nuts and seeds (Ch. 4) or with sprouts (Ch. 5).

## Chakra 5

1. Live food salads using all raw vegetables. Olive (or other) oil, onion, garlic, chili and radish make it a lower vibration meal. Also any form of seasoning such as Bragg or sea salt.
2. Green leaf and sprout salads with avocado or sprouted nut and seed dressings or avocado.
3. Nut and seed cheeses (fermented food) can be eaten with the vegetable or sprout salad provided avocado is not eaten.  Eat in moderation, they are acid-forming. Alternatively eat sprouted nut and seed salad dressings and dips.

4. *A high Ch. 5 food is a vegetable purée or juice; the more greens, the higher the vibration. You can add lemon if it makes it more palatable for you. Have an avocado on the side with it if you feel hungry. An example of a vegetable purée would be: juice of two lemons, three tomatoes, two carrots, a little red pepper, cilantro (or parsley or any other herb), spinach (or other greens), two celery stalks, one avocado. Blend.*

## Chakra 6

1. *Fruit*
2. *Fruit juices*
3. *Fermented vegetables*

*Most people have overdone sugar, carbohydrates and fruit in their life, so green juices are better than fruit juices. If you feel you do fine on fruit, have fruit juices but have the green juices too or mix the green juices with citric juices (See To To Life! by Artimia Arian for green juice examples). Always dilute the fruit juices with 50% or more water. Also have wheatgrass or other green drinks (with lemon and water if you can't stomach them neat). Blue-green algae is a good food for this chakra (if you do well with it) and Robert Young's Inner Balance is too or any other good green powder ( you can make your own by dehydrating and then dry blending a variety of green leaves).*

## Chakra 7

*Wheat or barley grass juice or any green juice.*

**✳✳✳✳✳✳✳✳✳✳✳✳✳✳✳✳✳✳✳✳✳✳✳✳✳✳✳✳✳✳✳✳✳✳✳✳**

*Powders such as cayenne pepper, and onion and garlic powder have a higher vibration than the vegetables. Thus, if you have digestive problems with onion, garlic or chili, try the powders.*

# *Protein*

*Extreme thinness is an indication of protein interference. The mechanical and chemical absorption of all you ingest, can be reduced by as much as 50%, which would naturally cause people to become excessively thin. One of the main reasons of poor nutrient absorption is because the small intestine (the location of food absorption) can be covered by Y/F symptogenic overgrowths. They displace the normal flora (the friendly bacteria which aids in the digestion and absorption of food elements). Robert Young estimates that over 50% of the U.S. populating is digesting and absorbing less than 50% of what they eat. (Sick and Tired, Robert Young).*

*Without proper nutrition the body is unable to heal and regenerate the body tissues. If the energy level is low and the regenerating capabilities are diminished for a period of time, naturally it follows that the aging process is accelerated.*

*Without protein and other essential nutrients, the body is unable to reconstruct tissues, especially muscle. It is also unable to produce enzymes, hormones or hundreds of other chemical components necessary for cell energy and organ activity.*

*Protein – soybean, lentil, tofu, raw seeds (sesame, sunflower, flax, pumpkin), raw nuts. Soaking nuts, seeds, legumes and grains for 12-24 hours before eating releases enzyme inhibitors, partially digests the protein, facilitating the digestion.*

*Ideas to increase protein consumption, while simultaneously working to devolve Y/F populations that are impeding protein and other nutrient absorption:*

1. *Dairy products and eggs (only if transitioning, try and substitute with soy and other products as soon as you are emotionally ready). The best dairy products are fresh yoghurt and cheeses, not milk or yellow cheeses.*
2. *Lentils – Soak the lentils overnight, pour off the water in the morning and allow them to sprout before using. Lightly steamed lentil sprouts (only steam for 5-10 minutes, they are much easier on the digestion and taste the same or better than boiled lentils).*
- *Lentil soup with lightly steamed or unsteamed lentil sprouts – add chopped tomato, onion, cilantro (celery, cucumber or other herbs or vegetables) and season with lemon, kelp, cayenne (oil, dulse or other seasoning). Same dish can be created with mung, alfalfa or any other sprouts or sprout mixtures or sprouts and greens. The broth can be created with juiced vegetables added to the water you used to sprout the lentils.*
- *Lentil sprout crackers – blend with onion, tomato (other vegetables and seasoning) and dehydrated.*
- *Lentil burgers – blend lentil sprouts with some carrots. Add chopped onion, cilantro, celery and red pepper, mix. Spread a little olive oil on the teflon pan with a paper serviette, heat the pan, place a tablespoonful of your mix, flattening it well and keep the pan on low heat. When the edges of your burger are nicely browned, flip it, thus cooking both sides. Do not place more oil for the remainder of the batch, simply scrape the pan well with your plastic egg flipper.*
3. *Tofu – Vegetable stir fry with tofu. (Refer to Tashirat Recipe Book for many quick and easy tofu dishes).*
4. *Nuts and seeds.*
- *Nut/seed milks - Blend nuts and seeds of choice well, strain with fine strainer. Heat if desired on low flame. Add Stevia to taste.*
- *Nut/seed crackers (dehydrated) with tomato, onion, kelp or other vegetables or seasoning.*

- *Nut/seed burgers (see Tashirat Recipe Book by Tashirat staff).*
- *Sesame or sunflower seeds lightly toasted. Gomasio – sesame seeds lightly toasted and dry blended with sea salt. Nut/seed powders, dry blended. For a sweet nut powder blend almonds and pecans, half and half. The powders can be sprinkled on a variety of dishes or eaten alone.*
- *Nut butters – Dry blend almonds or almonds and pecans and add grape seed or any other cold-pressed oil of your choice.*
5. *Dishes with mushroom, eggplant, nopal (See Chakra Recipe Guide by Artimia Arian).*
6. *Sprouts – soybeans, garbanzos, alfalfa, sunflower, sesame, lentils, mung.*
- *Steamed sprouted legumes especially garbanzo sprouts to make hummus. Healthier would be live garbanzo sprouts to make hummus. Blend garbanzo sprouts with lemon, oil, onion, garlic, celery. Blend till smooth. You can add red pepper. For cooked hummus dish sautee the onion and garlic (if desired) and add tahini. Burgers with any of the above.*
- *Any sprouts or live vegetables with nut/seed dressings or dips (To Life or Tashirat Recipe Book).*
7. *Purées – puréed sweet shakes (nut shakes) or soups (blended with vegetables and/ or herbs: sprouts, soaked or sprouted nuts/seeds, avocadoes) eaten slightly heated on a very low flame or at room temperature. Puréed lentil sprouts, tomato, onion, oil, cilantro, celery. The same with any other sprout or other vegetables. (Always put the tomato in the blender first so that everything blends easily.)*
8. *Greens – in salads, juices or green powders (purchased or home-made). For
Green powders, a good concentrated mineral powder which can be sprinkled on all foods, dry the greens of choice in the dehydrator or sun and then dry blend to a fine powder. Use a mineral chart to determine which greens*

*you would like to use. Greens in vegetable juices or vegetable purées.*

# Protein Transition

## Chakra 1

*Setas (large mushrooms) have a 1.5 vibration.*

## Chakra 2

*Eggs; natural yoghurt and fresh cheeses; cooked legumes; eggplant and mushrooms.*

## Chakra 3

*Tofu; soy meat.*

## Chakra 4

*Lightly sprouted and steamed legumes (lentils, garbanzos, soybeans); nuts and seeds; nut butters; dehydrated nut and seed or legume crackers; Brussel sprouts, broccoli, nopales and other high protein green vegetables; soy milk.*

## Chakra 5

*Sprouted nuts and seeds; nut and seed dressings or patés; nut and seed milks; sprouted legumes; sprouted legume soups or purées; whole, pureed or juiced greens (with vegetables).*

## Chakra 6

*Fermented nut/seed cheese; green juice with 2 or 3 tomatoes; green fruit smoothies.*

## Chakra 7

*Wheatgrass or barley juice; orange, apple or any high vibration fruit juice with green leaves.*

# Carbohydrates

*"The presence of complex and simple carbohydrate does not necessarily cause yeast or fungal overgrowths directly, but does promote a favorable environment for that which has evolved to grow more rapidly." (Sick and Tired, p. 42, Dr. Robert Young)*

*Transitioning off sugars:*

1. *Eliminate all sugar, refined products, molasses, cane sugar, honey. Substitute with Stevia, although even Stevia should be used in moderation.*
2. *Eliminate or reduce all starches (bread, tortilla, tubers such as potatoes, cooked grains, flour pastas). Eliminate or reduce all cooked sweet vegetables such as sweet potato, carrot, peas, beet, and pumpkin. Eliminate or reduce dried fruit and very sweet fruits such as bananas. Once the above have all been completely eliminated, move on to step 3.*
3. *Eliminate or reduce fruit. Once all fruit has been eliminated move to step 4.*
4. *Eliminate or reduce steamed and dehydrated vegetables. Once all steamed vegetables have been eliminated and you are able to eat a live food diet comfortably, move on to step 5.*
5. *Eliminate or reduce raw jicama, carrot and red pepper.*
6. *Eliminate or reduce all nuts and seeds unless sprouted or soaked.*
7. *Eliminate or reduce tomato and avocado.*

*Although this is applicable to patients, in particular those with Candida and other yeast or fungal overgrowths, it is most significant for spiritual aspirants who are in ascension and exposed to high Cosmic Energy. For the carbohydrate content of foods, it is best to check mineral charts. Ann Wigmore provides good ones in The Blending Book and The Hippocrates Diet, however, bear in mind that the carbohydrate content of vegetables is for raw vegetables. It increases considerably when they are cooked.*

# Blended Foods for Easy Digestion

Read:

- *The Sunfood Cuisine by Frederic Paténaude*
- *The Blending Book by Ann Wigmore and Lee Pattinson*

## Guidelines for Live Food Blending Soup Meals

*Always chop the tomato and put it in the blender first, in addition to any liquids, to help facilitate the blending. These recipes can be done without added liquid but add water (or cucumber) if wanting a thinner consistency. You can use a variety of vegetables juiced rather than water to blend the vegetables – mineral-rich organic water. By using less water and more watery vegetables, less seasoning needs to be added, if any at all.*

*All raw food recipes can be very slightly heated on a low flame – use a teflon pan. Add more of any vegetable or less according to your liking.*

*To all recipes add lemon, oil, kelp, cayenne or any herbs and seasoning of choice. You can use celery and high sodium greens, such as Swiss chard or any other, rather than sea salt. Don't use too many sweet vegetables such as carrot, beet, jicama and red pepper but use them in moderation to sweeten the dishes when needed. Add finely chopped herbs if needed before serving. Be creative.*

1. *Use non-sweet fruits as the liquid soup base. Blend them first and then add the other ingredients. Examples:*

*tomatoes, cucumber, tomatillos (green, yellow), green or red pepper, zucchini. Vegetable juice can also be used as a base.*

2. *For consistency add: nuts and seeds (always soaked), avocado, lentil or other legume sprouts (garbanzo, soy beans), olive oil (or other cold-pressed oil).*

3. *Add any vegetables and greens of choice: asparagus, broccoli, green beans, spinach etc.*

4. *Add any vegetables or ingredients as condiments: cayenne, kelp, dulse flakes or other sea vegetables, sea salt (Bragg, miso, tamari sauce etc.), chives (use the green leaves too), onion, garlic, chili peppers, curry powder, ginger.*

5. *Almonds – soak overnight, place in a little nearly boiling water for 5 to 10 seconds. Run cold water over them immediately and remove the shells.*

6. *Add more or less liquid vegetables or purified water according to the desired consistency. Add herbs (basil, thyme, cilantro, parsley) etc. and other condiments to taste.*

7. *All recipe examples provided are for one serving and are but a basic guideline for you to make your own soups quickly and easily. For many more ideas and recipes read the recommended books, and experiment.*

*Blend:*

1. *1 large tomato, two celery stalks, lentil sprouts, onion and cilantro to taste.*

2. *2 avocados, cilantro, lemon, spinach, cucumber.*

3. *1 tomato, garbanzo sprouts, lemon, oil, onion, garlic, celery.*

4. *1 tomato (and or cucumber), soaked almonds and pecans (or other nuts and seeds), broccoli (or asparagus or any other vegetable of choice), parsley.*

# Live Food High Protein Soup Example

## Lentil Soup

3-4 tomatoes (or more for thinner soup)
2 handfuls of sprouted lentils
cayenne, kelp, chives etc. to taste

## Broccoli Soup

5-6 tomatillos
½ head and stalk (peeled) of broccoli
2 handfuls of almonds (always soaked and shelled)
chives, cayenne, (Bragg, garlic, etc.)

## Asparagus Soup

4 tomatoes
2 handfuls of sunflower seeds (soaked)
10-15 stalks of asparagus
juice of two lemons
condiments

If protein is not a concern, use avocado blended with vegetables.

# Steamed Vegetable Soup Examples

Steam and blend, putting watery vegetables like zucchini or tomatoes in the blender first for easy blending. Add steamed tomatoes and cayenne or any other chili for a heavier soup.

**Note:** The hotter the soup, the lower the vibration. The more chili, steamed tomato, garlic or onion, the lower the vibration (and the reverse). You know the person needs a low vibration if they say they need heavy food.

## Zucchini or Chayote

Blend alone with any other vegetable such as steamed or raw tomato.

## Cauliflower

Blend alone, has taste and consistency of mashed potato. Add a very little water to blend.

Blend with a very few zucchinis.

Use zucchini and cauliflower soup as a smooth creamy base for any other soups.

## Broccoli or Chayote

Blend with almonds and chili.

# Nut or Seed Milks

*Almonds are best soaked and shelled. One or two handfuls of nuts/seeds per glass of water. Blend and strain. Reuse the pulp in your next nut/seed drink. Top with cinnamon. They can be blended with apple (remove skin), papaya, mango or other fruit if no digestive problems.*

# Nut or Seed Butters

*Dry blend almonds, pecans or any other nuts or seeds of your choice. Add grape seed oil or any other cold-pressed oil to make a nut butter. Almonds with oil work well. Almonds and pecans with oil work well.*

# The New Era

The Cosmos is emerging from an era of extreme negativity and unconsciousness to an era of ultra positivity and consciousness. To emerge from the comatose state we have all lived in to lesser and greater degrees, healthy balanced lifestyles and diet are crucial. The higher one's diet, the clearer one's mind and the more naturally spiritual and less material we become.

This nutritional knowledge is specifically for those on a spiritual path, ascending from a grosser material vibration to a higher subtler spiritual vibration. Food is a more powerful tool than most people realize. One has to experiment with it to realize its power, so be aware of what you do. Transitioning is always preferable. It is so important to always take the emotional body into account, especially regarding food, as food is most people's comfort zone. So avoid inflexible disciplinary measures, gradually transition over time, keeping the emotional body happy. No dietary regime will benefit the physical body if the emotional body is not kept comfortable and happy.

For evolution (growth) to be enduring and permanent, it needs to be a thorough process; it's not an overnight affair. A tree that shoots up too fast, will have a weak root system and trunk, and will not endure. It's the tree that grew steadily over time, with the well-developed roots and thick trunk that will weather all storms.

# An Important Note To Readers

June 2014

Dear Readers,

Recently I was introduced to Dr. Graham's 80-10-10 diet. I need to express how fully I endorse it as a Chakra 5 and 6 diet, if that is appropriate for your current life lessons. All of my nutrition books can be used as a transition to Dr. Graham's diet, which is a pure Chakra 5 & 6 diet. The more greens and non-sweet vegetables one consumes, the more it is a Chakra 5 diet. The more sweet fruit, the more it would fall into a Ch. 6 diet category.

All of the nutrition knowledge in my books must therefore please be modified, reducing the fat intake to achieve an 80-10-10 ratio ideally or no more than 30% fat initially as you are reducing. As raw foodists, we have all erroneously over-consumed very high fat foods such as cold-pressed olive oil, nuts and seeds and avocados. To give you an idea: if you consume approximately 2000 calories a day, ideally you should not consume more than 100g of an avocado a day (a third of a medium to large avocado), OR the equivalent of 15 almonds, OR 1 tbs. of olive oil. If you raise your caloric intake, then you would be able to eat more fat and more protein. The important thing is that your ratio approximates the ideal 80-10-10. You can accumulate these quantities - eat no fat for a three days and then eat an avocado in the evening with your salad.

There is a very simple website – www.nutridiary.com – that calculates the percentages of your daily caloric food intake. I really advise you to get someone to teach you the basics of how to use the site, which would take no more than a half an hour class at the most. If you don't know anyone to teach it to you, Tashirat can

send you an instruction video. Write us your request to the email listed at our website: (www.tashirat.com).
If you find it too challenging to transition to the 80-10-10 diet alone, we can help you with consultations in person or by e-mail. Just contact us and we'll gladly help you. We also offer nutrition courses, which include Yoga, Meditation and Chakra classes.

To conclude, anyone interested in nutrition needs to read Dr. Graham's outstandingly simple, clear and informative 80-10-10 book. I wish I would have found it 30 years ago but the book only came out in 2008 and I was only introduced to it very recently. I'm in 100% agreement with all that he so eloquently and concisely imparts in his valuable book. One cannot expect emotional, mental and spiritual body health and happiness (balance), without achieving physical body health.

Dr. Graham's book has to be supplemented by all of my nutrition books, which are essential as they focus on vibrational nutrition.

To Health, Love and Life!

With love,
Artimia

*p.s. I do not personally know Dr. Douglas Graham, but from over a year of experience on ourselves, our Tashirat children and students we find the 80/10/10 diet that Dr. Graham promotes invaluable as a Chakra 5 & 6 diet.*

*If transitioned correctly, fully taking into consideration the person's vibration, evolution and present physical condition, the 80/10/10 diet is excellent information.*